Adaptive Sports for the Disabled

Your Guide to Accessible Activities and Events

Table of Contents

Chapter 1. Introduction

Welcome to a world where barriers dissolve and limitations are liquidated! This Special Report titled "Adaptive Sports for the Disabled: Your Guide to Accessible Activities and Events," prides itself on embodying the spirit of true possibility. Delve deep into the heart of accessibility as we curate a comprehensive collection of adaptive sports and events that cater to the diverse aspirations of those with disabilities. We're thrilled to introduce you to inspiring individuals, groundbreaking organizations, and transformative support systems that are changing lives and shaking up misconceptions. This report will not only educate you but will also inspire you to take action, put your game face on, and experience the indomitable strength of human will. Build your confidence, boost your motivation, and broaden your horizons - there's a whole world of adapted sports waiting for you! So, are you ready to gracefully vault over the trivial constraints of disability? Your journey into the exhilarating realm of adaptive sports begins here! Get your copy now and let the games begin!

Chapter 2. Empowering Through Sports: An Introduction to Adaptive Sports

The human spirit is indomitable, boundless, and forever in search of platforms that allow it to freely express its virtues and capabilities. For individuals with disabilities, this assertion is no less valid or potent. Recognizing this, the arena of adaptive sports have, over the years, grown to become a place where barriers dissolve into inconsequence, limitations liquidate into oblivion, talents emerge triumphant, and resilience triumphs.

2.1. The Genesis of Adaptive Sports

The genesis of adaptive sports can be traced back close to a century, to the period following World War II. It was the war veterans with disabilities who first took the initiative to engage in sports activities as a form of rehabilitation. Consequently, sport began to be recognized not only as a medium for physical therapy but also as a means of social reintegration. Over time, certain adaptations were made to traditional sports to make them more accessible for those with disabilities, thus birthing the concept of 'adaptive sports'.

These sports are about tailoring the activity to the participant. Sports that were hitherto seen as insurmountable for individuals with disabilities were adapted and modified. Equipment was remodeled, rules were tweaked, and structural changes were made to ensure that those with different strengths and abilities could passionately participate and compete.

2.2. The Broad Spectrum of Adaptive Sports

The range of adaptive sports currently out there is impressively broad and diverse. It spans from team sports like wheelchair basketball, wheelchair rugby, and blind soccer, to individual events such as wheelchair tennis, adaptive golf, and adaptive sailing.

Team sports typically involve structural and rule-based modifications that allow for an equal field of competition for all participants. For example, in wheelchair basketball, points may be awarded based on the player's classification, which is a measure of their functional abilities, in order to level the playing field.

In individual sports like adaptive golf, modifications may involve changes to equipment and rules. For instance, the use of specialized golf clubs and carts that allow the player to strike the ball from a seated position, or permitted exceptions to certain rules, like movement of the ball.

2.3. The Impact Beyond the Playing Field

Apart from physical benefits such as improved mobility, strength, and coordination, the impact of adaptive sports extends well beyond the playing field. Firstly, they foster social inclusions by bringing together individuals from diverse backgrounds and abilities to interact, compete, and imbibe from one another's experiences.

The sense of camaraderie nurtured through these sports has important psychological implications such as improved self-esteem and confidence. By focusing on ability rather than disability, they also shift the public's perception of individuals with disabilities from being seen as recipients of care, to be recognized as agile participants in the game of life.

Moreover, involvement in sports often leads to improved academic and employment outcomes. The discipline, teamwork, and perseverance learned on the playing field translate beneficially to different aspects of daily life including school and work.

2.4. Towards a More Inclusive Future

Looking towards the future, the adaptive sports movement is increasingly promoting inclusion where individuals with and without disabilities play on the same team. This move is believed to cultivate empathy, acceptance, and understanding, while providing a level playing field that celebrates individual capabilities over traditional notions of sports prowess.

In a nutshell, adaptive sports open the doors to an exciting world where physical boundaries are erased and spirits are enkindled with newfound vigour. They are about celebrating extraordinary performances under extraordinary circumstances. They are about defying odds, challenging conventions, and sculpting champions out of the 'can'ts' and 'won'ts'. And at the crux of it all, they uphold the indubitable truth that sports, as a universal language, has the power to evoke change, transform perceptions, and above all, to empower.

As you embark on this exploration of adaptive sports, remember, this world isn't about 'making the best of a bad situation', but rather about exploiting the abundant opportunities that lie therein. And as you navigate through it, witness its transcending power that has the potential to change lives and the way we perceive disability, forever.

So here's an invitation to delve further into the world of adaptive sports, to unmask the champions, unearth the grit, and understand the transformative power of sportsmanship that prevails in this realm. Whether you're a spectator, a participant, or an enthusiast, you're part of a movement that is redefining the landscape for individuals with disabilities, one dribble, one stride, and one victory at a time. Welcome to the world of adaptive sports!

Chapter 3. Breaking the Barriers: The Evolution of Adaptive Sports

The landscape of physical activity has significantly evolved over time, opening up limitless possibilities for individuals with differing abilities. This evolution is not just about the sports themselves, but about a revised perception of disability, driving societal change, and fostering inclusion.

3.1. The Genesis of Adaptive Sports

What we see today as a vibrant, energizing and inclusive sporting ecosystem for people with disabilities had humble beginnings. The genesis was simple yet powerful: the desire to empower, and the need to break away from societal constraints. But where and when did adaptive sports originate?

The earliest records of structured, competitive sports for people with disabilities date back to the aftermath of World War II. With numerous veterans and civilians left with physical and psychological disabilities, there was a dire need to help these individuals reintegrate into society and rebuild their lives. The role of Sir Ludwig Guttmann, a neurologist at the Stoke Mandeville Hospital in England, was instrumental in using sports as a form of physical therapy. In 1948, he organized a competition for wheelchair athletes, which in many ways mirrored the Olympics.

3.2. Wheelchair Basketball and the Paralympics: Sports See a Radical Shift

Guttmann's competition was a key catalyst in the formation of the Paralympic Games, a worldwide multisport event for athletes with disabilities. Coinciding with the 1960 Summer Olympics in Rome, the first official Paralympics was held, opening a new chapter in the world of adaptive sports.

In the same period, another significant development was the formation of the National Wheelchair Basketball Association (NWBA) in the USA in 1949. Founded by World War II veterans, it was the first association dedicated to promoting and developing a single, specific adaptive sport on a large scale.

Wheelchair basketball paved the way for the realization that any sport could be adapted, leveling the playing field for people with disabilities.

3.3. Expansion of Adaptive Sports in the Late Twentieth Century

With the solid foundation provided by the Paralympics and organizations like the NWBA, the latter half of the century saw a surge of adaptive sports. This was a time of innovation and expansion, leading to the inclusion of new sports like wheelchair rugby, boccia, and goalball in the Paralympics.

Sports, formerly inaccessible for people with disabilities, evolved to accommodate them. The physically demanding sport of rugby was adapted into wheelchair rugby (initially called murderball due to its aggressive, high-collision nature) for quadriplegic athletes. Goalball was specifically designed for visually impaired athletes, utilizing tactile and auditory senses instead of sight. Boccia emerged as a precision ball sport similar to lawn bowls, specifically designed for athletes with more severe physical disabilities.

3.4. Adaptive Sports in the Twenty-First Century: A New Dawn

Today, adaptive sports incorporate virtually any sporting activity - skiing, sailing, basketball, fencing, and even dancing. The inclusion of technology has revolutionized adaptive sports, making them more accessible and competitive. Be it specially-designed sports wheelchairs, prosthetics for running, or electronic devices to aid visually impaired athletes, technology has certainly given adaptive sports a new dimension.

Sporting organizations for people with disabilities have blossomed, providing opportunities for active participation in adaptive sports at grassroots, national, and international levels. Events like the Invictus Games and the Special Olympics World Games highlight the global recognition and acceptance that adaptive sports have garnered.

3.5. The Impact of Adaptive Sports on Society

Adaptive sports have not just been transformative for those directly involved, but also have had a profound impact on society as a whole. Beyond providing opportunities for physical activity, they challenge the wild misconceptions, promote social inclusion, and forge stronger, more understanding communities.

The journey of adaptive sports - from its initiation as a form of rehabilitation for war veterans to becoming a global phenomenon - communicates a powerful message of resilience, courage, and the breaking of barriers. Society's perception of 'disability' has been significantly challenged and altered, with a new focus on abilities rather than the lack thereof.

In conclusion, the evolution of adaptive sports reflects a broader cultural, social, and technological evolution. It is a decisive shift away from perceiving disability as a limitation towards acknowledging and celebrating differing abilities in the sporting arena. As we look ahead, we see adaptive sports at the forefront of driving further societal change, using the power of sport to emphasize ability over disability, pushing boundaries, and continuously breaking barriers.

Chapter 4. Profiles in Adaptability: Inspiring Athletes in the Adaptive Sports Community

The world of adaptive sports showcases a panorama of human endurance and determination, where athletes with disabilities continually affirm their tenacity. This chapter unveils inspiring stories and profiles some of the most remarkable athletes who are redefining the very essence of sportsmanship.

4.1. Barrier Breakers: Bold and Brave

A host of athletes reach out to the adaptive sports community, each with a unique story of challenge, transformation, and triumph.

Leading the brigade is Sarah Reinertsen, the first female leg amputee to complete the Ironman World Championship. Facing the amputation of her left leg at the tender age of seven, Sarah turned her tale of adversity into one of strength, growing into a world record holder, author, motivational speaker, and model for athletes worldwide.

Next up is Tatyana McFadden, born with a rare form of spina bifida leaving her paralyzed from the waist down. Despite the odds, her spirit never faltered. She's a decorated Paralympian with dozens of medals across summer and winter sports. Named one of the most influential people in the world by the Time magazine, Tatyana continues to captivate hearts across the globe.

4.2. Paralympic Powerhouses: Lighting the Path

The Paralympics offer a grand stage for athletes with disabilities. Here we encounter individuals such as Matt Stutzman, also known as the Armless Archer. Born without arms, Matt has mastered the art of shooting arrows using his feet. Winning a silver medal at the 2012 Paralympic Games, Matt truly encapsulates the notion 'disability is not inability.'

Then there's Jessica Long, a double lower-limb amputee who has swum her way to become one of the most decorated Paralympians in history. With 23 medals to her name, Jessica inspires with her relentless determination and fierce competitive spirit.

4.3. All About Adaptation: Innovators in Action

From basketball to rock climbing, a diverse array of adaptive sports figures reflect the unlimited scope of human potential.

Dylan Alcott, an Australian wheelchair basketball and tennis player, advocates for people with disabilities. A victim of a tumor in his spinal cord, Dylan embraced his disability with aplomb, earning gold medals in both sports. He is also a radio host, a TV personality, and a motivational speaker.

Similarly, Hugh Herr, despite losing both his legs due to frostbite, is a renowned rock climber and biophysicist. He has designed his prosthetic legs to enable a level of climbing competitiveness that surpassed his pre-amputation abilities.

4.4. Beyond Borders: Global Inspirations

The landscape of adaptive sports is global, with athletes challenging societal norms and advocating inclusivity.

South Africa's Oscar Pistorius, known as 'Blade Runner' due to his prosthetics, challenged the traditional athletic narratives by racing in both Paralympic and Olympic competitions.

Another inspirational figure is Monoluck Skywalker, a Cambodian landmine survivor and marathoner. His determination to compete and win against non-disabled athletes has made him a powerful advocate for disabled rights in South East Asia.

The lives and stories of these adaptive athletes serve not only as testimonials of human spirit and willpower; they are also a call to action – an invitation to each of us to recognize that each hurdle can be leaped, each challenge can be overcome, and each dream can be realized.

Adaptive sports continue to break new ground in the realm of disability, redefining 'impossible' and unveiling the extraordinary capabilities within each of us. These inspiring tales of courage and determination iterate that barriers can be overcome, limits can be surpassed, and dreams are there for the taking, no matter the circumstances.

Chapter 5. Sport for All: Understanding Different Adaptations for Various Disabilities

Adaptive sports, sometimes known as Parasports, refer to both competitive and recreational sports designed for athletes with disabilities. These adaptive athletic activities act as platforms where limitations are abolished, and every aspiring athlete, regardless of their disability, can participate and excel.

5.1. Life Beyond Limitations

In the realm of sports, physical challenges do not dictate an athlete's potential. Assisting people with disabilities and mobility challenges, adaptive sports provide an avenue for participation where once there were barricades. Whether it's through a sport as intense as wheelchair rugby or as graceful as seated dancing, adaptive sports has made its mark through many barriers, serving as a champion of inclusivity.

In the subsequent sections, we'll work our way through a variety of common disabilities, delving into the modifications and accommodations made within different sports to ensure they're accessible and enjoyable for everyone.

5.2. Physical Disabilities

Physical disabilities encompass a broad spectrum of conditions and impairments. A key element of ensuring fair and enjoyable competition is the classification system. Athletes are grouped based on their functional ability, ensuring that everyone competes on a level playing field.

1. `Spinal Cord Injuries`: Wheelchair sports such as basketball, rugby, and racing have been adapted for athletes with spinal cord injuries. Modifications such as specially designed wheelchairs and adjusted rules promote full engagement in these sports.

2. `Amputations`: Prosthetics and other assistive technology enable athletes with limb loss or limb difference to participate in a variety of sports, from running and cycling to swimming and skiing.

3. `Cerebral Palsy`: Sports such as boccia and CP football have specific rules and classifications for athletes with cerebral palsy. Standing frames, assistive throws, and adapted sports equipment are frequently used.

5.3. Visual Impairments

People with varying degrees of visual impairment compete in many adaptive sports. The sports are often modified using auditory cues, tactile feedback systems, and guides to help athletes navigate the activity.

1. `Goalball`: Exclusively for athletes with visual impairments, goalball relies on sound indicators within the ball to facilitate gameplay.

2. `Judo`: Athletes with visual impairments participate in judo competitions unmodified due to the tactile nature of the sport.

3. `Paratriathlon`: Paratriathlon uses guide runners and tactile signaling systems to make the sport accessible to athletes with visual impairments.

5.4. Hearing Impairments

Individuals with hearing impairments compete in almost every sport at both elite and recreational levels. Technological adaptations and visual signaling systems allow athletes to communicate and interact.

1. `Deaf Basketball`: Accommodations such as illuminated shot clocks and visual signals instead of whistles make the sport more accessible to players with hearing impairments.

2. `Skiing`: Vibrating vests and visual signaling systems are used to communicate with athletes during downhill and cross-country skiing.

5.5. Intellectual Disabilities

Contrary to popular assumption, having an intellectual disability isn't a barrier to participating in a wide array of sports, thanks to accommodations aimed at simplifying rules and improving understanding.

1. `Special Olympics`: This global organization provides training and competitions in a variety of sports for athletes with intellectual disabilities.

2. `Unified Sports`: In these sports, athletes with and without intellectual disabilities compete alongside each other, promoting social inclusion and breaking down barriers.

5.6. Power of Adaptive Devices and Assistive Technologies

Advancements in adaptive devices and assistive technologies have played a pivotal role in making sports more accessible to persons with disabilities. Beyond just the provision of custom-made wheelchairs and artificial limbs, we're talking about technologically advanced prosthetics that allow for natural running motion, sports wheelchairs designed for speed and agility, and sensory devices that assist visually impaired athletes.

Recapping, adaptive sports are not just about recreation. They provide an opportunity to enhance physical ability, lift self-esteem, and foster social inclusion, prompting a transformative change in an individual's lifestyle. Acknowledging this significance, we realize the impact that each adapted sport has on people with disabilities. It is indeed 'Sport for All,' bringing everyone together on the same playing field, proving that the perceived obstacles to involvement in sports are indeed surmountable.

The world of adaptive sports is endlessly evolving, constantly pushing the boundaries of what is possible and paving the way for even more people to partake in the joy and camaraderie of sport. Armed with knowledge, understanding, and the right attitude, we can all become active participants in this sporting revolution.+

Chapter 6. Game-Changing Innovations: Adaptive Equipment and Technological Advancements

Breakthroughs in technology have been breaking down barriers for individuals with disabilities, allowing them to engage in sports and physical activities that were once deemed impossible. As we navigate through this section, we'll explore some of the game-changing, adaptive equipment and highlight key technological advancements that have redefined the landscape of sports for the disabled.

6.1. Power of Personalized Prosthetics

Modern prosthetic technologies have made leaps and bounds over what was previously available. Traditional prosthetics are often heavy, inflexible, and awkward for sports. However, innovations in materials and design have led to lighter, more flexible solutions that not only replace missing limbs but also enhance athletes' abilities in their chosen sports.

For instance, running blades, pioneered by companies like Össur and Otto Bock, are tailored to provide the perfect blend of responsiveness and flexibility for sprinters, enabling athletes to achieve remarkable speed and agility. Similarly, Touch Bionics' prosthetic hands offer unparalleled dexterity, enabling athletes to participate in sports that require intricate hand movements.

In the arena of water sports, companies such as Northwell Health have been trailblazers in developing swim-specific prosthetics. Their innovation, "The Fin," is a 3D-printed, amphibious, prosthetic leg that provides a vastly improved swimming experience for amputees.

Moreover, companies such as UNYQ are revolutionizing prosthetics by making them personalized. They offer a wide range of customizable designs that not only adapt to the needs of their users but also align with their personal identities making the prosthetics an extension of their personalities.

6.2. Revolutionizing the Wheel: Advances in Wheelchairs

One of the most significant areas where technology has revolutionized adaptive sports is in the realm of wheelchairs. These advancements have not only enhanced general mobility for athletes but have allowed participation in an expanding array of sports.

In wheelchair basketball, products like Per4max are allowing athletes to move and maneuver with ease and efficiency. With lightweight shock-absorbing frames, they provide players with unparalleled speed and agility.

Progress has been equally promising on the rugby field. Products like the Quickie All Court Sports Wheelchair, known for its lightweight design, aluminum framing, and superior maneuverability, have given athletes the necessary speed and agility to perform aggressive, lightning-fast moves during games.

Furthermore, innovations aren't just limited to the court. The GRIT Freedom Chair, an all-terrain wheelchair, has transformed outdoor exploration, enabling individuals to traverse hiking trails, sandy beaches, and more.

Perhaps the most remarkable innovation in this field is the powered wheelchair, like the StrikeForce by Quantum Rehab. This high-performance power wheelchair allows a whole new level of participation in sports, with its superb acceleration, top-end speed and safety measures.

6.3. Technological Infusion: Wearable Tech & Virtual Reality

With the advent of wearable technology and virtual reality (VR), athletes with disabilities are breaking new grounds. Wearable tech, like fitness trackers and smartwatches, enable athletes to monitor their training, track their progress and fine-tune their strategies.

Meanwhile, companies such as eSight are changing lives by harnessing the power of VR. eSight's eyewear uses a high-speed, high-definition camera to capture everything the user looks at, and algorithms enhance the video feed, which is then projected onto screens in front of each eye. This allows legally blind individuals to participate in various sports.

Notably, VR is also being used for therapeutic purposes. BreakAway VR is a program designed to help wheelchair users improve their mobility skills in a risk-free environment. This sort of technology could revolutionize rehabilitation, giving individuals a safe space to develop confidence and refine their abilities.

6.4. The Future is Accessible

While we have already witnessed a huge transformation in adaptive sports due to technology, future advancements hold even more promise. Exoskeleton technology could provide a revolutionary way for individuals with paralysis to stand, walk, and even run in marathons. Similarly, advancements in AI could lead to 'smart' prosthetics and wheelchairs, further enhancing their adaptability and effectiveness.

Moreover, as the global emphasis on inclusivity intensifies, investment in adaptive sports technologies is likely to grow, leading to more cutting-edge breakthroughs. The possibilities are vast and only limited by our imagination.

These innovations in adaptive sports technology are not just improving physical possibilities; they are also breaking down societal barriers and reshaping perspectives regarding disability. As this evolution continues, we will undoubtedly reach a future where everyone, regardless of their physical condition, can participate - and excel - in the sport they love.

Chapter 7. Diving into Inclusion: Exploring Global Adaptive Sports Events

We begin our exploration at the epicenter of adaptive sports, the Paralympic Games. Since its inaugural event in 1960, the Paralympics have been the beacon of inclusivity, showcasing the extraordinary abilities of athletes with disabilities on a global stage. The Paralympics host a multitude of sports, each adapted to accommodate the needs of the courageous athletes who defy the odds to participate in this monumental celebration of human strength and perseverance.

7.1. The Paralympic Phenomenon

The Paralympics provide an unparalleled platform for athletes with a range of disabilities to compete in conventional sports, modified to ensure fair and accessible competition. The classifications, often based on the type and severity of the disability, help to ensure a level playing field. Let's take a look at some of the high-profile adaptive sports events featured in the Paralympics.

1. Seated Volleyball: Introduced in the Netherlands in the 1950s, seated volleyball made its Paralympic debut in 1980. It is the same classic game, but with a few adaptations, including a smaller court and a lower net. Here, all players' sitting bones must be in contact with the floor when they hit the ball.

2. Goalball: Invented in 1946 to rehabilitate visually impaired World War II veterans, Goalball took the Paralympics stage in 1976. Eliminating the element of sight, teams of three use their bodies and ears to block a ball that rings as it rolls.

3. Paracanoeing: Paddling on to the Paralympic scene in 2016, this

sport welcomes athletes with physical and visual impairments to navigate sprint routes. Modifications include sitting or kneeling positions, and choices between single or double-bladed paddles.

7.2. Special Olympics: A Spotlight on Unified Sports

If there's one event that exemplifies the spirit of inclusion, it is the Special Olympics. Established in 1968 by Eunice Kennedy Shriver, the Special Olympics has grown to support over 5 million athletes in 172 countries. Unified Sports, a key part of the Special Olympics, is an inclusive sports program that brings together athletes with and without intellectual disabilities to train and compete on the same team.

From the exciting game of Bocce, where teams strategize to throw balls closest to a smaller ball called 'pallina,' to the popular Unified Basketball, where athletes of diverse abilities integrate seamlessly - the Special Olympics perpetuates Shriver's vision of fostering a world of acceptance and inclusion via sports.

7.3. Invictus Games: Heroes Embodying Invincible Spirit

Founded by Prince Harry, the Invictus Games is a multinational sports event for wounded, injured, and sick military personnel and their associated veterans. Introduced in 2014, it's not the medals or awards athletes compete for here but the unyielding spirit, the resilient camaraderie, and the victorious personal achievements.

Featuring adaptive sports like wheelchair basketball, sitting volleyball, and indoor rowing, the Invictus Games salute the unwavering spirit of servicemen and women, symbolizing the unbreakable will of the true warriors of our time.

7.4. Regional Adaptive Sports Events

Region-specific events are equally important in championing the cause of adaptive sports, reaching out to corners of the globe the larger events may not penetrate. Asia Pacific's Arafura Games, Canada's Canada Games, Europe's IWAS Games, all offer platforms for the differently-abled to shine. They foster localized networks of athletes and trainers to uplift the adaptive sports scene from the grassroots level.

7.5. The Thrill of Adventure: Beyond the Competitive Arena

Besides structured sports events, numerous organizations invite people with disabilities to break free from stereotypes and embrace adventurous pursuits. Organizations like Adaptive Adventures and Disabled Sports USA offer adventure sports like rock climbing, water skiing, mountain biking, and snowboarding – all tailored for individuals with disabilities.

In this tapestry of global adaptive sports events, everyone can find their spot under the sun. Sports that were once inaccessible have now been redefined and adapted, making them inclusive and inviting to all. This journey paints a picture of progress and resilience, showing us that the human spirit knows no bounds! Whether it's about competing on a global platform or embracing the thrill of an adventure sport, the choice is now yours to make. The world of adaptive sports awaits you!

"The only limits you have are the limits you believe." - Wayne Dyer

Chapter 8. Local Opportunities: Finding Adaptive Sports Events Near You

Embracing the universe of adaptive sports introduces you to a wealth of opportunities just around the corner. Discover ways to locate events and connect with organizations offering adaptive sports in your local vicinity.

8.1. Scouring Your Locale

Begin by exploring your own surroundings, which is as simple as searching the internet or asking around in your community. Various resources are at your fingertips, including local newspapers, community billboards, and online platforms dedicated to informant about local sports events. These can provide a wealth of information about any upcoming adaptive sports events. Make a note of regualr event schedules, entry requirements, and the sports offered.

8.2. Connecting with Local Adaptive Sports Organizations

Depending on your location, there might be numerous organizations that facilitate adaptive sports for individuals with disabilities. By getting in touch with these organizations, you can gain insights about the sporting events they host and join a like-minded community. Some well-known adaptive sports organizations include Adaptive Sports USA, Disabled Sports USA, and Paralympic Sports Clubs. However, there might be smaller, local groups too that operate in your city or state.

Let's take a look at some ways to discover these organizations:

- **Online Directories:** Browse through the websites and directories of bigger associations such as Adaptive Sports USA, Disabled Sports USA, or the American Association of Adapted Sports Programs. They often include a list or a map of their registered local affiliates, making it easier to find an approachable organization near you.

- **Local Community Centers or Recreation Departments:** Many community centers and recreation departments offer adaptive sports programs. Make use of the resources provided on their websites or visit them in person to gather information.

- **Rehabilitation Centers and Hospitals:** Medical facilities offering rehabilitation services might also have connections with local adaptive sports organizations. They serve as a great resource for discovering sports events and activities.

- **Social Media:** Social media platforms, particularly Facebook groups or Instagram pages, can serve as a great avenue to reach out to local organizations or groups. Searching for adaptive sports in your area on these platforms might lead you to communities of enthusiastic individuals pursuing various sports.

8.3. Catering to Your Interests

Once you've identified the local organizations and resources available, the next step is to find events that cater to your specific interests. This largely entails considering your preferred type of sport - whether it's a physically intense game like wheelchair basketball, a mind sport like chess, or a calm and relaxing activity such as adaptive yoga. Each adaptive sports organization will likely cater to a wide array of interests and abilities, so take the time to ascertain which events best suit your preferences.

8.4. Engage in Volunteering

Interestingly, another enlightening perspective to the adaptive sports world is through volunteering. Local sports organizations often need volunteers to support their operations. This could be anything from assisting athletes, setting up facilities, coordinating logistics, or even spreading the word about their events. Volunteering is more than just giving a helping hand. It provides an inside look, ground level insights, and a profound understanding of adaptive sports.

8.5. Networking with Adaptive Athletes

Building connections and networks never fails. Spend time chatting with other adaptive athletes in your area. Their personal experiences in the local sport scene can provide valuable, timely, and precise information that's hard to find otherwise. These networks, both online and offline, are the veins and arteries of adaptive sport ecosystems.

With these strategies and resources, you're now equipped to explore the local adaptive sports ecosystem and discover remarkable events and activities. The journey towards adaptive sports is thrilling, enlightening, empowering - and it all starts with information. Let this guide serve as a compass to navigate you along your journey. And remember, adaptive sports isn't just about the game; it's about embracing a fuller life, transforming your mindset, and inspiring others along the way. Through adaptive sports, breaking barriers and overcoming limitations are just another part of the game. Take the first step, gear up, and step into the vast, welcoming arena of adaptive sports.

Chapter 9. Moving Boundaries: The Role of Advocacy in Adaptive Sports

Advocacy – both collective and individual – has proven instrumental in the journey towards reduction of barriers and inclusion in adaptive sports. It is through the relentless voices of advocates that constructive dialogues are initiated, stigmas are confronted, and much-needed changes in policy and practices are effected.

9.1. The Power of Advocacy

Advocacy is essentially about championing for a cause, stimulating change, and driving improvements through assertive, informed actions. It denotes empowering individuals, communities, or interest groups to assert their rights and create a conducive environment to foster their interests.

When harnessed in the realm of adaptive sports, advocacy has remarkable potential. It can amplify the voices of those with disabilities, leading to the creation of transformative narratives about their abilities rather than focusing on their limitations. This compelling storytelling can go a long way in challenging misconceptions, evoking empathy, and igniting public interest, lying the groundwork for systemic change.

Advocates, whether they are persons with disabilities, their families and friends, role models, or compassionate activists, play a crucial role in influencing public opinion and shaping policies. By highlighting the benefits of adaptive sports – the joy, camaraderie, and empowering effect it can have – these advocates essentially transform societal lingering stereotypes about disabilities. However, it's not an easy fight, and it involves challenging the status quo and navigating opposition; but the rewards, both collective and individual, are profound.

9.2. Shaping Policy through Advocacy

Policy advocacy is a powerful tool for bringing about widespread changes. It involves influencing the decision-making processes at various levels, pushing for policies that are inclusive, accommodative, and align with the interests of the adaptive sports community.

A classic example of successful policy advocacy is the enactment of the Americans with Disabilities Act (ADA) in 1990 and its subsequent influence worldwide. By outlawing disability-based discrimination and mandating reasonable accommodations, this groundbreaking policy thrust open many previously closed doors to a variety of sports and recreational pursuits for the disabled. The ADA laid the groundwork for other similar laws around the globe that seek to promote inclusivity and equitable access in sports.

These fruitful endeavours demonstrate how relentless and coordinated advocacy can result in favourable policy changes. Moreover, these instances highlight the transformative potential of policy, underscoring why concerted efforts towards influencing policy are a key weapon in the advocacy arsenal.

9.3. Advocacy and Accessibility

Advocacy has played a large role in enhancing accessibility to adaptive sports, be it the availability of sports facilities, the accessibility of equipment, or the opportunities for participation and competition. Advocates have tirelessly worked to create partnerships with stakeholders, conduct outreach programs, and increase funding options for adaptive sports.

For instance, the endeavours of organizations like Disabled Sports USA, The National Center on Health, Physical Activity and Disability (NCHPAD), and the Adaptive Sports Foundation have been instrumental in promoting accessibility to sports for people with disabilities.

These organizations tactfully combine advocacy and action, working towards inclusivity not only by pushing for changes in policies but also by directly creating inclusive spaces, funding adaptive equipment, and facilitating training and participation in various sports.

9.4. Advocacy, Representation, and Visibility

One major area where advocacy has proved vital is the domain of representation and visibility. Despite the myriad benefits of adaptive sports, the representation of disabled athletes in mainstream media is disproportionately low.

Advocates across the world strive to address this gap. They work towards boosting the visibility of athletes with disabilities, showcasing their achievements, their challenges, and stories. This visibility is crucial to inspire individuals with disabilities, empowering them to break barriers that have held them back.

Such representation careers an important space in societal consciousness, creating new paradigms of what is possible and redefining 'limitations.' Further, it helps sensitize society, leading to increased recognition of the abilities of those with disabilities and fostering a more accepting and inclusive community.

In conclusion, advocacy is a crucial enabler in the realm of adaptive sports. It takes the baton of empowerment, striving ceaselessly to dissolve boundaries, transform narratives, and create a world where everyone has the freedom to pursue their sporting dreams. Advocacy for adaptive sports is advocacy for equal opportunities, representation and rights – it's a call for seeing beyond disabilities, towards abilities and possibilities. This fight for empowerment and inclusivity will continue to intensify and expand, moving boundaries and inspiring action in the coming times.

Chapter 10. Staying Fit, Having Fun: Adaptive Sports for Health and Wellness

Physical fitness and wellness ought to be a prime consideration for everyone – disabled or not. In this section, we explore an array of adaptive sports tailored to cater for various disabilities, crisscrossing the territories of physical exertion, mental stimulation, social connections, and therapeutic advantages.

10.1. Overcoming Obstacles: The Importance of Adaptive Sports

Participation in sports has always been one of the most engaging ways to keep fit, maintain a sound mind, and live healthily. Everyone, irrespective of their physical abilities or limitations, should have access to the tremendous benefits sports offer. Adaptive sports, also known as para sports, are modified versions of traditional sports or entirely new sports specifically designed for people with disabilities - a true manifestation of strength, endurance, and courage.

Engagement in adaptive sports not only serves the purpose of facilitating physical fitness, but it also bolsters emotional wellness by fostering feelings of inclusion, motivation, and self-esteem. In addition, participation in these sports cultivates social connections, teamwork, and relationships, all the while annihilating the societal prejudices that surround disability.

10.2. The Wide Spectrum of Adaptive Sports

The arena of adaptive sports is incredibly diverse, offering numerous choices for individuals of all abilities. Here's a look at some of the most popular adaptive sports.

10.2.1. Wheelchair Basketball

One of the most recognized adaptive sports is wheelchair basketball. Integrating the speed, agility, and skill of traditional basketball, it offers athletes with physical disabilities an exciting avenue for competitive sport. Special rules, such as considering a push on a wheelchair equivalent to steps taken while running or walking, ensure fairness and inclusivity.

10.2.2. Adaptive Rowing

For those drawn to water, adaptive rowing can be both therapeutic and challenging. Adaptive rowing offers a low-impact but high-intensity workout that ripples through every muscle in the body. Special equipment like fixed seats or chest straps are used to accommodate athletes with disabilities.

10.2.3. Goalball

Designed specifically for athletes with visual impairments, Goalball takes the hearing sense to an entirely new level. Athletes try to throw a bell-equipped ball into the opponent's net while the opposing team attempts to block the ball. It serves as an excellent way to improve spatial awareness and auditory skills.

10.3. Accessible Fitness: Powering Health Through Adaptive Sports

While competitive adaptive sports vastly contribute to physical well-being, fitness-focused adaptive activities also hold great value in promoting health and wellness. These activities aim to constructively align physical and mental wellness elements into a neat balance.

10.3.1. Adaptive Yoga

Adaptive Yoga modifies traditional yoga postures for individuals with mobility issues. It creates a welcoming and accessible environment for individuals who may feel excluded from traditional yoga classes. Props such as blocks, straps, or chairs help adapt each pose to the individual's unique capabilities.

10.3.2. Wheelchair Aerobics

Wheelchair aerobics offer individuals with mobility impairments a chance to boost heart rates, improve cardiovascular health, and strengthen muscles. The exercises can range from low to high intensity, featuring rhythmic movements, resistance training, and stretch routines.

10.3.3. Handcycling

Handcycling is an excellent workout for people with limited lower body mobility. It strengthens the upper body, improves cardiovascular function, and offers a refreshing way to enjoy the outdoors. From recreational biking to competitive racing, handcycling is a versatile adaptive sport.

10.4. Choosing the Right Adaptive Sport

The choice of an adaptive sport significantly depends on an individual's interests, physical capabilities, availability of local resource and training programs, and the possibility of participation in group activities. Seeking advice from health and physical education professionals can lend a substantial hand in this decision-making process.

10.5. Adaptive Sporting Events

Remarkable international, national, and local events are held annually where adaptive athletes compete and showcase their abilities. Notable among these includes the Paralympics, the Special Olympics, and the Invictus Games. Such tournaments not only provide a platform for the athletes but also promote awareness and acceptance of disability sports worldwide.

In conclusion, adaptive sports offer an avenue towards achieving fitness, fun, and excellent health while hammering out the societal norms surrounding disabilities. Whether you're playing for leisure, health, or competitive thrill, the onus is on enjoying your chosen sport to the extent that even the process of participation outweighs the outcome. So, gear up, take your pick, and bask in the exhilarating world of adaptive sports! Life is your playground, and every challenge a game – let's play!

Chapter 11. Your Next Steps: Getting Involved in the Adaptive Sports Community

Congratulations! By making it this far, you've already taken the first step towards joining the active and passionate community of adaptive sports. However, the journey is far from over. Here, we will provide you a comprehensive set of steps to enter, thrive, and make your mark in this incredible world.

Getting involved with adaptive sports is much more than just participating in activities; it's about belonging to a community of likeminded people who are breaking barriers and shattering stereotypes every day.

11.1. Finding Your Fit

The inaugural step in your adaptive sports journey is finding your perfect fit. With the vast array of adaptive sports available for people with various types of disabilities, you're sure to find the right one for you. You may already have a sport in mind, perhaps one you have enjoyed pre-disability, or maybe the excitement of exploring something completely new is more appealing.

Participating in adaptive sports comes with great physical benefits. According to research, regular physical activity decreases the risk of a range of health issues including heart disease, diabetes, and obesity. Additionally, endorphin release from physical activity is known to reduce stress, anxiety, and depression.

Remember, there are no right or wrong choices here, and it's perfectly okay to try a few different sports before settling on your favorite. Consider the resources you have available around you, including local adaptive sports clubs, and what physically suits you best.

11.2. Connecting with Local Organizations

Once you've found a few possible sports, connect with local organizations, clubs, and facilities that offer programs for adaptive sports. These organizations can furnish you with greater detail about what you need to get involved, including sport-specific equipment, practice schedules, and the support they provide to help you participate comfortably and confidently.

Adaptive sports organizations offer various levels of activity, from recreational to professional, so you can find a comfortable starting point and aspire for gradual progression. Many organizations offer adaptive-specific coaching and mentorship opportunities, and can point you towards grants, scholarships or other financial aids to get you going.

11.3. Acquiring the Right Equipment

Most adaptive sports require specialized equipment tailored to the needs of athletes with disabilities. While this may seem intimidating and costly, many organizations provide rental equipment or have programs designed to help new athletes manage these costs. There are grants and funding programs available that can alleviate the financial burdens of acquiring necessary sports equipment.

Do ample research and ask around in your new community, as many athletes sell or donate their used equipment when they upgrade. Plus, many manufacturers and pro shops offer discounts to athletes competing at a semi-professional or professional level.

11.4. Testing the Water

Once you have the necessary equipment, it's time to hit the field, court, track, or pool. Start slow, get comfortable with the equipment, and don't push yourself too hard right from the start. Take advantage of any training sessions your local organization might offer.

Most adaptive sports programs will encourage you to come and try their sport for free first. They often have 'come and try' days or 'rookie days' targeted at introducing new participants to the sport in a fun and non-competitive environment. Learn from experienced facilitators at these events, and don't hesitate to ask questions.

11.5. Enhancing Your Skills

Once you've found the sport you love and you're comfortable with all the moving parts, it's time to focus on improving your skills. Whether your aspirations lean towards professional competition or you're more interested in taking part for fun, remaining dedicated to improvement will heighten your experience and satisfaction.

Consider hiring a dedicated coach or trainer to help you focus on skill improvement. Participate in skill development workshops and clinics. Immerse yourself in your chosen sport and learn from watching professional athletes, reading relevant literature, and obtaining feedback from peers and coaches.

11.6. Growing into the Community

A significant benefit of adaptive sports is the community that comes with it. As you participate more, attend events, and increase your involvement, you'll naturally find a place within the vibrant community of participants, volunteers, families, and supporters. Engage in social events and volunteer opportunities – they are plentiful within this supportive environment.

In closing, stepping into the world of adaptive sports requires some planning, commitment, your effort, and yes, a leap of faith. However, as you take each step, you'll find yourself increasingly enriched by the experience. The road ahead is certainly promising and exciting, so go ahead, take the plunge and make your adaptive dream come true. There is an extraordinary journey waiting for you in the world of adaptive sports, and you're more than capable of embracing it. Let the games begin!